KNOWLEDGE GUIDE TO
CARPAL TUNNEL SYNDROME

Comprehensive Guide To Symptoms, Treatment, Prevention, And Pain Relief Techniques For Wrist Health

DR. AARON BRANUM

Copyright © 2024 BY DR. AARON BRANUM

All rights reserved. Except for brief quotations embodied in critical reviews and certain other noncommercial uses permitted by copyright law, no part of this publication may be reproduced, distributed, or transmitted in any form or by any means, Including photocopying, recording, or other electronic or mechanical methods, without the prior written permission of the publisher.

Disclaimer:

The data in this book, is solely meant to be informative and instructional.

This book is not intended to replace expert medical advice, diagnosis, or care. No medical, health, or other professional services are offered by the author, publisher, or any affiliated parties

Individual outcomes may differ in the practice of these therapies, which entail a variety of approaches and methodologies.

A one-on-one session with a trained or certified healthcare professional is still preferable. It is best to consult a trained healthcare provider before making any decisions regarding your health.

The author of this book is not affiliated with any specific website, product, or organization related to any of these therapies.

All reasonable measures have been taken by the author and publisher to guarantee the authenticity and dependability of the material contained in this book.

Contents

CHAPTER ONE 13

  CARPAL TUNNEL SYNDROME (CTS): WHAT IS IT? 13

    An Explanation And Definition Of CTS 13

    Anatomy Of The Carpal Tunnel And Wrist .14

    Reasons And Danger Factors For CTS 14

    Day-To-Day Effects Of CTS 16

CHAPTER TWO 17

  UNDERSTANDING DIAGNOSIS AND SYMPTOMS 17

    Common CTS Symptoms 18

    Tests And Procedures For Diagnosis 20

    Setting CTS Apart From Other Conditions .21

    The Value Of Seeking Medical Guidance ... 23

    Talking About Symptoms With Medical Experts 24

CHAPTER THREE 27

  MEDICATION OPTIONS: FROM SURGICAL TO CONSERVATIVE 27

    Non-Surgical Methods For Treating CTS ... 27

Pain And Inflammation Medications 29

Surgical Procedures In
More Serious Situations 30

CHAPTER FOUR 35

CHANGES IN LIFESTYLE AND PREVENTIVE
MEASURES 35

Tips For Ergonomics To Avoid CTS...........35

Stretching Activities For Healthy Wrists....36

The Significance Of Hand Position And
Posture...36

Modifications To Lifestyle To Lower CTS Risk
....37

Establishing A Handle-Friendly Workplace.38

CHAPTER FIVE 39

COPING MECHANISMS AND SELF-CARE
METHODS 39

Controlling Soreness And Pain At Home ...39

Self-Massage Methods For Relieving Wrist
Pain 40

Stress Reduction For Patients With CTS....40

Including Methods Of Relaxation 41

5

The Value Of Self-Care In The Management Of CTS 42

CHAPTER SIX 43

MEDICAL THERAPY AND REHABILITATION .. 43

Physical Therapy's Role In CTS Recovery .. 43

Exercises To Increase Flexibility And Strength In The Wrist 45

Programs Of Rehabilitation For Patients With CTS 46

Collaborating With A Physical Therapist 48

Long-Term Advantages Of Rehab 49

CHAPTER SEVEN 53

FOR CTS, ACUPUNCTURE AND ACUPRESSURE 53

Spinal Alignment And Chiropractic Care ... 55

Supplements And Herbal Remedies 57

Talking About Alternative Therapies With Medical Professionals 60

Complementary Therapies: Including Them In CTS Treatment Plans 62

CHAPTER EIGHT 67

TIPS FOR DAILY ACTIVITIES FOR PEOPLE LIVING WITH CTS 67

Modifications For Typical Daily Tasks 67

Utilizing Assistive Technology In CTS Management 68

Advice For Operating A Vehicle, Typing, And Other Tasks 69

Activity And Rest Balanced For Healthy Wrists 70

Asking Friends And Family For Support 71

CHAPTER EIGHT 73

PROSPECTIVE DEVELOPMENTS AND STUDIES IN CTS MANAGEMENT 73

New Approaches To Treat CTS 73

Progress In Diagnostic Methods 76

Studies On The Prevention Of CTS 79

CONCERNING THIS BOOK

For anyone struggling with or trying to understand this common but sometimes misdiagnosed ailment, the "Knowledge Guide to Carpal Tunnel Syndrome" is an invaluable resource.

Its exhaustive inquiry commences with a detailed examination of the complexities of Carpal Tunnel Syndrome (CTS), providing a precise definition and clarifying the structure of the wrist and carpal tunnel.

Through an exploration of the causes and risk factors, the guide highlights the value of early diagnosis and treatment, giving readers a critical basis upon which to understand the need for proactive management.

A crucial part of the process is comprehending symptoms and diagnosis, which equips readers with the skills necessary to identify typical CTS symptoms and complete diagnostic procedures. With this information at hand, readers can converse with healthcare providers in an informed manner, opening the door for prompt intervention.

Additionally, the book skillfully traverses the spectrum of available treatments, from conservative methods to surgical procedures, each supported by a careful analysis of advantages and disadvantages.

Furthermore, the handbook goes beyond therapeutic approaches to include lifestyle modifications and preventative actions, emphasizing the significance of ergonomic habits, stretches, and the creation of an atmosphere that is wrist-friendly. It emphasizes the value of holistic self-care by providing coping mechanisms and self-massage methods that enable people to proactively manage their pain and suffering.

The adventure continues with an emphasis on physical therapy and rehabilitation, illuminating the revolutionary role that exercises and rehabilitation programs play in improving wrist flexibility and strength.

To promote a comprehensive approach to the therapy of CTS, alternative and complementary therapies are also examined. Readers are provided with a range of possibilities, including acupuncture, chiropractic care, and herbal remedies.

Everyday life tips are like a lighthouse, providing modifications for everyday chores and methods for finding the right balance between work and relaxation.

The handbook offers optimism for future developments that could completely change the field of CTS management by shedding light on new trends and research directions. Essentially, the "Knowledge Guide to Carpal Tunnel Syndrome" goes beyond the typical confines of a simple educational tool and becomes a source of empowerment and knowledge for everyone affected by this illness.

CHAPTER ONE

CARPAL TUNNEL SYNDROME (CTS): WHAT IS IT?

Carpal Tunnel Syndrome (CTS) is a prevalent ailment affecting the wrist and hand that results in tingling, numbness, and discomfort. It happens when there is compression or squeezing of the median nerve at the wrist, which passes from the forearm into the hand.

An Explanation And Definition Of CTS

Put more simply, CTS is the result of compression or squeezing of the median nerve at the wrist, which supplies feeling to the palm side of the thumb, fingers, and little finger only. The hand and wrist experience discomfort, tingling, numbness, and weakness as a result of this compression.

Anatomy Of The Carpal Tunnel And Wrist

A basic understanding of the anatomy of the wrist and carpal tunnel is necessary to comprehend CTS more fully. The wrist's carpal tunnel is a small opening created by ligaments and bones. Both the tendons and the median nerve that regulates finger mobility pass through this tube. CTS symptoms are caused by pressure on the median nerve, which occurs when the tissues around the wrist flexor tendons enlarge or the tunnel narrows.

Reasons And Danger Factors For CTS

The emergence of CTS can be attributed to various circumstances. One typical cause is repetitive hand and wrist movements, especially when done forcefully or in an awkward position. Inherited medical disorders that can raise the chance of getting CTS include diabetes, obesity, and rheumatoid arthritis. Hormonal shifts, such as those brought on by pregnancy or menopause, can also make a person more susceptible to CTS.

The Value of Prompt Identification and Intervention

To stop additional damage and relieve symptoms, it is essential to diagnose and treat CTS as soon as possible. Ignoring symptoms or postponing treatment can exacerbate discomfort, numbness, and weakness, making day-to-day tasks more difficult. Seeking medical attention as soon as possible is essential for accurate diagnosis and the successful application of treatment plans that may involve splinting, medication, lifestyle adjustments, ergonomic adjustments, or, in extreme circumstances, surgery.

Day-To-Day Effects Of CTS

CTS can have a major influence on day-to-day functioning, making it difficult to do basic tasks like typing, holding objects, and even buttoning clothes.

CTS-related pain, numbness, and weakness can make daily tasks uncomfortable and challenging, including working.

Moreover, the negative effects of CTS on general well-being may be worsened by sleep disturbance brought on by nighttime symptoms.

Maintaining quality of life and reducing disruption from CTS requires good management through appropriate treatment and lifestyle modifications.

CHAPTER TWO

UNDERSTANDING DIAGNOSIS AND SYMPTOMS

Several symptoms can indicate compression of the median nerve within the wrist's carpal tunnel, which is the cause of carpal tunnel syndrome (CTS). Frequently, these symptoms begin gradually and get worse with time. Tingling or numbness in the thumb, index, and middle fingers is a typical early symptom. This could feel like it goes up the arm. Forearm, wrist, and hand pain are common symptoms of CTS, and they frequently get worse at night. Muscle atrophy brought on by nerve compression can also result in hand weakness and a propensity to drop objects.

Healthcare practitioners use a variety of clinical examinations and testing to appropriately diagnose CTS. These include Phalen's maneuver, in which holding the wrist flexed exacerbates symptoms, and Tinel's sign, in which tapping over the median nerve causes tingling or shock-like sensations. Furthermore, nerve conduction studies (NCS) and electromyography (EMG) can detect compression points and evaluate nerve function. To view the structures inside the wrist and find any anomalies, imaging methods like magnetic resonance imaging (MRI) or ultrasound may be used.

Common CTS Symptoms

Understanding the typical signs and symptoms of carpal tunnel syndrome (CTS) is essential for prompt diagnosis and treatment. A common sign is tingling or numbness in the thumb, index, and middle fingers, which frequently spreads to the forearm. When engaging in repetitive wrist motion activities, such as typing or using portable gadgets, this sensation, called paresthesia, may get worse. CTS patients may also have hand weakness, which makes it difficult for them to grip objects or use their fine motor skills.

Pain or discomfort in the forearm, wrist, or hand is another defining sign of CTS. The degree of this discomfort can range from minor to severe, and it can be made worse by particular actions or postures, including sleeping with the wrist bent forward. Symptoms that occur at night are very prevalent and might interfere with sleep cycles. If left untreated, CTS can cause the affected hand's muscles to weaken and atrophy, which can impair dexterity and coordination.

Tests And Procedures For Diagnosis

Several clinical evaluations and specialized tests are used to diagnose carpal tunnel syndrome (CTS), which is the diagnosis of median nerve compression within the carpal tunnel. Electromyography (EMG) is a frequently employed test that quantifies the electrical activity of muscles in response to nerve stimulation. The strength and speed of nerve signals as they pass through the carpal tunnel are also assessed by nerve conduction studies (NCS). These examinations aid in identifying nerve malfunctioning sites and assessing the severity of CTS.

Healthcare practitioners may use physical examinations in addition to electrodiagnostic tests to look for telltale indicators of CTS, like Tinel's sign and Phalen's maneuver. Tapping the median nerve at the wrist to cause tingling or shock-like feelings in the fingers is known as Tinel's sign. On the other hand, Phalen's maneuver involves reproducing CTS symptoms by holding the wrist flexed. To see the internal structures of the wrist and find any structural anomalies causing nerve compression, diagnostic tests such as magnetic resonance imaging (MRI) or ultrasound may also be suggested.

Setting CTS Apart From Other Conditions

To accurately diagnose and treat carpal tunnel syndrome (CTS), it is necessary to distinguish it from other disorders that present with similar symptoms.

Even though tendonitis, arthritis, and peripheral neuropathy are similar to CTS, there are some clinical indicators and diagnostic procedures that can help distinguish between the three. For example, numbness and tingling in the thumb, index, and middle fingers are common symptoms of CTS and might exacerbate at night or during certain tasks requiring wrist flexion.

When differentiating CTS from other neuropathic disorders, electrodiagnostic techniques such as nerve conduction studies (NCS) and electromyography (EMG) are essential.

These examinations evaluate the median nerve's health and function and assist in locating any compression or dysfunction within the carpal tunnel. Physical investigations that replicate symptoms of median nerve compression, such as Tinel's sign and Phalen's maneuver, can also help in the clinical diagnosis of CTS.

The Value Of Seeking Medical Guidance

When experiencing symptoms that could indicate carpal tunnel syndrome (CTS), it's critical to consult a doctor as soon as possible for the best course of action. Even while at first modest symptoms could be controlled with rest and lifestyle changes, if CTS is left untreated, it can worsen and cause chronic discomfort, weakness, and impairment of hand and wrist function. Early diagnosis enables medical practitioners to treat patients appropriately and stop additional nerve damage.

Furthermore, only licensed healthcare providers are capable of doing the specific clinical evaluations and diagnostic procedures needed for an appropriate diagnosis of CTS. Postponing medical examinations can lead to chronic pain and a slower rate of healing. People who feel they may have CTS should consult a doctor right away so they can obtain timely therapies, including physical therapy, corticosteroid injections, or splinting, to relieve symptoms and enhance hand function.

Talking About Symptoms With Medical Experts

Accurate diagnosis and treatment of carpal tunnel syndrome (CTS) depend on open communication with medical providers. It's critical to be as specific as possible when discussing symptoms with a healthcare professional, including the start, length, and course of symptoms as well as any triggers or mitigating variables. Furthermore, providing pertinent medical history—such as past injuries or underlying illnesses—can aid in directing the diagnosis and therapy suggestions.

Healthcare providers may conduct diagnostic tests and physical examinations during the consultation to look for evidence of median nerve compression and rule out other possible reasons for the patient's symptoms.

By communicating any changes in their symptoms or how their treatments are working, patients can take an active role in their diagnosis. Healthcare professionals may customize treatment programs to each patient's needs and improve carpal tunnel syndrome patients' outcomes thanks to this cooperative approach.

CHAPTER THREE

MEDICATION OPTIONS: FROM SURGICAL TO CONSERVATIVE

Compression of the median nerve in the wrist can result in Carpal Tunnel Syndrome (CTS), a disorder that can cause discomfort and limit the movement of the hand and wrist. Depending on the severity of the symptoms and the specifics of each case, treatment options for CTS might range from conservative approaches to surgical techniques.

Non-Surgical Methods For Treating CTS

Particularly in milder cases, non-surgical treatments are frequently the first line of defense against carpal tunnel syndrome. These methods, which do not require intrusive procedures, concentrate on discomfort relief and inflammation reduction.

Braces or wrist splints are a frequent non-surgical treatment for CTS. By maintaining the wrist in a neutral position, these devices can lessen symptoms like pain and tingling and relieve strain on the median nerve.

An additional non-surgical alternative for treating CTS is occupational therapy. A licensed occupational therapist can assist people in determining whether ergonomic problems at work or in their everyday routines are causing or exacerbating their symptoms. To increase wrist flexibility and strength, they might also offer stretches and exercises.

Making changes to one's lifestyle can also be very helpful in controlling CTS symptoms. This can mean staying away from activities that make symptoms worse, like typing for extended periods or using a computer mouse or wrist motions that are repetitive. Reducing symptoms can also be achieved by implementing ergonomic changes to workstations and employing appropriate hand and wrist placement when performing tasks.

Pain And Inflammation Medications

Medication may occasionally be recommended to assist in controlling the discomfort and inflammation brought on by CTS. It could be advised to use nonsteroidal anti-inflammatory medications (NSAIDs) like naproxen or ibuprofen to lessen discomfort and swelling.

For those with CTS, injectable corticosteroids are an additional treatment choice. Some patients have quick symptom relief from these injections because they directly administer potent anti-inflammatory medication to the afflicted location.

It's crucial to remember that although drugs may be useful in treating symptoms, they are usually not a long-term fix for CTS. They are frequently used with other non-surgical procedures to offer short-term comfort while longer-term options are investigated.

Surgical Procedures In More Serious Situations

Surgical surgery may be required for those with severe or persistent CTS symptoms who do not respond to non-surgical therapy.

The most popular surgical treatment for carpal tunnel syndrome (CTS) is carpal tunnel release surgery, which includes releasing the transverse carpal ligament to relieve pressure on the median nerve.

Open surgery and endoscopic surgery are the two primary methods used in carpal tunnel release surgery.

The transverse carpal ligament can be immediately accessed by the surgeon during open surgery by making a tiny incision in the hand's palm. With endoscopic surgery, the surgeon is guided through a smaller incision with the use of specialized instruments and a tiny camera, perhaps leading to less tissue damage and a quicker recovery period.

Restoring hand function and reducing symptoms of carpal tunnel syndrome can be achieved with both open and endoscopic carpal tunnel release surgery.

But as with any surgical operation, there are possible risks and side effects to take into account, including infection, nerve damage, and wrist stiffness.

advantages and disadvantages of various treatments

The advantages and disadvantages of any treatment option for carpal tunnel syndrome should be carefully considered.

For many CTS sufferers, non-surgical treatments like wrist splints, occupational therapy, and medication can be quite effective and low-risk.

Surgical intervention can be required, nevertheless, if the symptoms are severe or do not improve with non-surgical therapy. Carpal tunnel release surgery includes some hazards, including infection, nerve damage, and wrist stiffness, even though it is quite efficient at reducing symptoms and restoring hand function.

In the end, seeking non-surgical or surgical treatment for CTS should be decided after consulting with a trained medical professional. They can assist people in comprehending their options, balancing the advantages and disadvantages, and creating a treatment strategy that is specific to their requirements and situation.

CHAPTER FOUR

CHANGES IN LIFESTYLE AND PREVENTIVE MEASURES

Tips For Ergonomics To Avoid CTS

By making sure that your workspace is optimized for both comfort and efficiency, ergonomics plays a critical role in preventing Carpal Tunnel Syndrome (CTS). To maintain a neutral wrist position while typing or using a mouse, start by adjusting your workstation and chair.

Your wrists should not be overly twisted up or down; they should be straight. Think about making an ergonomic mouse and keyboard purchase to encourage a more comfortable hand position. To further lessen shoulder and neck pain, place your display at eye level.

Stretching Activities For Healthy Wrists

Frequent stretches can increase the range of motion and lower the risk of CTS. To release tension in the wrist and forearm muscles, perform basic wrist stretches throughout the day, such as wrist flexor and extensor stretches.

To increase circulation and lessen stiffness, you can also include workouts that concentrate on the hand and finger muscles. To preserve balance and avoid asymmetries that may exacerbate CTS, always remember to stretch both sides equally.

The Significance Of Hand Position And Posture

It's crucial to keep your wrists in the proper position and with proper posture to avoid CTS. When working, try not to slouch or lean forward since this might put more strain on your wrists and compress your median nerve. Rather, sit up straight, keep your elbows close to your torso, and your shoulders relaxed. To lessen the tension on the carpal tunnel, keep your wrists neutral, neither bent up nor down. Throughout the day, pay attention to your posture, whether you're working at a desk or doing other tasks.

Modifications To Lifestyle To Lower CTS Risk

You can lower your risk of CTS greatly by changing your lifestyle. If you use tools or type repetitively, for example, your wrists will get tired. Take regular breaks to stretch and rest your muscles. Try to stay away from tasks that require tight grips or strong wrist motions. To lessen strain on the carpal tunnel and adjacent structures, keep a healthy weight. Furthermore, if you smoke, give it up since it can worsen circulation and raise your chance of CTS.

Establishing A Handle-Friendly Workplace

Preventing CTS requires designing a work environment that is wrist-friendly. Make sure your desk is tidy and well-lit to reduce mess and distractions. To support your wrists when typing or using a mouse, utilize wrist rests or padding. To lessen the pressure on your hands and wrists, think about utilizing ergonomic equipment or speech recognition software. To avoid overuse injuries, encourage employees to rotate duties and take regular breaks. You may lower the risk of CTS and increase employee well-being by fostering a supportive work environment.

CHAPTER FIVE

COPING MECHANISMS AND SELF-CARE METHODS

Although carpal tunnel syndrome (CTS) can be difficult to live with, there are coping mechanisms and self-care practices that can assist in effectively managing the illness. These methods seek to enhance general well-being by reducing pain and discomfort.

Controlling Soreness And Pain At Home

Controlling pain and discomfort at home is essential to living with CTS. This can be accomplished in several ways, including by using ice packs on the injured wrist, taking over-the-counter painkillers like acetaminophen or ibuprofen, and employing wrist splints to support and lessen wrist strain. Furthermore, using proper posture and ergonomics when doing repeated wrist motion duties will help reduce problems.

Self-Massage Methods For Relieving Wrist Pain

Techniques for self-massage may also help relieve CTS-related wrist pain. The wrist and forearm muscles and tendons can be gently massaged to ease tension and increase blood flow. To release tight muscles and reduce discomfort, try kneading, circular motions, and light stretching. To prevent aggravating symptoms, it's crucial to be careful and not exert excessive pressure.

Stress Reduction For Patients With CTS

Using stress management strategies in daily life can assist manage CTS symptoms as stress can increase the condition's symptoms. Stress levels can be lowered and relaxation can be encouraged via methods including progressive muscle relaxation, deep breathing techniques, and meditation. Additionally, stress can be reduced and general well-being can be enhanced by partaking in joyful and relaxing activities like practicing hobbies, going on nature hikes, or listening to music.

Including Methods Of Relaxation

Relaxation methods can be incorporated into daily life to help control CTS symptoms in addition to stress management strategies. Exercises like tai chi, yoga, and moderate stretching can ease tension in the muscles, increase relaxation, and enhance flexibility. Additionally, by enhancing body awareness and posture, these exercises might lessen wrist strain and stop symptoms from getting worse.

The Value Of Self-Care In The Management Of CTS

Effective self-care is essential to controlling chronic tension syndrome. Taking care of oneself on a physical, mental, and emotional level can help reduce symptoms, enhance general health, and stop more issues. This includes using proper ergonomics, exercising frequently to build muscle and increase flexibility, getting enough sleep, and keeping up a nutritious diet. Additionally, since pushing through pain or discomfort can exacerbate symptoms, it's critical to pay attention to your body and take breaks when necessary. People with CTS can enhance their quality of life and effectively manage their condition by making self-care a priority and implementing healthy lifestyle practices.

CHAPTER SIX

MEDICAL THERAPY AND REHABILITATION

Physical Therapy's Role In CTS Recovery

An all-encompassing recovery plan for Carpal Tunnel Syndrome (CTS) must include physical therapy. It focuses on giving the injured wrist and hand their full range of motion, strength, and flexibility back. People with CTS can restore ideal hand and wrist health and address underlying issues that are contributing to their disease by working with a qualified physical therapist.

Reducing inflammation and pressure on the compressed median nerve, which is a main objective of physical therapy for CTS, is one of its main objectives. To reduce symptoms and encourage recovery, therapists employ a range of methods, including electrical stimulation, ultrasound, and manual treatment. With these procedures, the affected area's blood circulation is improved and discomfort and edema are reduced.

The use of customized exercise regimens is another essential component of physical therapy in the rehabilitation process for CTS. By strengthening the muscles that surround the wrist and hand, these workouts aim to improve stability and support for the afflicted joint.

Furthermore, certain stretches aid in increasing the range of motion and flexibility, which lessens the stiffness and discomfort that are frequently connected to CTS.

Exercises To Increase Flexibility And Strength In The Wrist

Those with Carpal Tunnel Syndrome (CTS) can greatly benefit from adding focused workouts to their everyday routine. By increasing wrist strength and flexibility, these exercises hope to relieve pressure on the median nerve and lessen the symptoms of CTS.

Wrist curls are a useful workout to strengthen your wrists. Hold a lightweight (such as a dumbbell or a water bottle) in your hand with your palm facing upward to complete this exercise.

Curl your wrist slowly up and back down to the beginning position. As your strength increases, gradually increase the weight as you perform multiple repetitions of this motion.

Wrist extension exercises are also effective. To begin, set your forearm down on a table or other level surface and hang your hand over the edge, palm down.

Raise and lower your wrist slowly while holding a small weight in your hand. This exercise strengthens and stabilizes the wrist joint by focusing on the muscles on the rear of the forearm.

Programs Of Rehabilitation For Patients With CTS

For individuals with Carpal Tunnel Syndrome (CTS), specialized rehabilitation programs are crucial to accelerating recovery and averting symptom recurrence in the future. A variety of interventions, such as physical therapy, ergonomic adjustments, and lifestyle modifications, are often used in these programs.

Education is a vital part of CTS rehabilitation programs. Along with learning how to manage their symptoms and stop additional aggravation, patients also learn about the underlying reasons for their ailment. Therapists offer advice on good body mechanics and workstation arrangements to lessen wrist and hand strain during daily tasks.

Furthermore, manual therapy techniques are frequently incorporated into rehabilitation programs to address soft tissue constraints and enhance joint mobility.

To relieve muscle tension and encourage relaxation in the affected area, therapists may use light stretching and massage techniques.

Collaborating With A Physical Therapist

To maximize the efficiency of rehabilitation efforts in the recovery of Carpal Tunnel Syndrome (CTS), cooperation with a qualified physical therapist is important. To address each patient's unique symptoms and functional constraints, therapists evaluate each patient's needs and create individualized therapy regimens.

To increase wrist strength, flexibility, and function, patients closely collaborate with their physical therapist throughout therapy sessions, carrying out recommended exercises and approaches. Therapists offer practical advice and constructive criticism to guarantee good form and technique, maximizing the advantages of every exercise.

Physical therapists frequently recommend at-home exercise regimens in addition to in-clinic sessions to enhance in-person therapy sessions. By enabling patients to carry out their rehabilitation activities on their own time in between sessions, these exercises hasten the healing process and promote long-term development.

Long-Term Advantages Of Rehab

Patients with Carpal Tunnel Syndrome (CTS) can benefit much in the long run from investing in rehabilitation.

Rehabilitation programs assist in enhancing general wrist and hand health by addressing underlying conditions that contribute to CTS symptoms, such as joint stiffness and muscle weakness.

A major long-term advantage of therapy is the decrease in CTS pain and discomfort.

Patients can reduce inflammation and relieve pressure on the median nerve by using focused exercises and manual treatment techniques. This will lower pain levels and enhance quality of life.

Rehabilitation also encourages functional restoration, which enables people with CTS to restore their capacity to carry out everyday chores more easily and effectively.

While flexibility exercises increase range of motion and joint mobility, strengthening exercises improve grip strength and dexterity, allowing patients to participate in activities they enjoy without any limits.

All things considered, enrolling CTS patients in a thorough rehabilitation program produces long-lasting outcomes, enabling them to live active, pain-free lives and reducing the likelihood of symptom recurrence.

Over time, people can effectively manage their condition and preserve good wrist and hand function by implementing ergonomic improvements, frequent exercise, and lifestyle alterations.

CHAPTER SEVEN

FOR CTS, ACUPUNCTURE AND ACUPRESSURE

Traditional Chinese medicinal methods including acupressure and acupuncture have drawn interest as possible cures for Carpal Tunnel Syndrome (CTS). Acupressure applies pressure to certain body areas, whereas acupuncture inserts tiny needles into predetermined locations. Both seek to balance the body's qi, or energy flow and encourage the body's natural healing processes.

Studies on the effects of acupuncture and acupressure on CTS patients have demonstrated encouraging outcomes in terms of reducing discomfort, tingling, and numbness in the hands and wrists. These methods might lessen pressure on the median nerve, which is frequently compressed in CTS, as well as lessen inflammation and enhance circulation.

A skilled practitioner will carefully place needles at specific places along the meridians—energy pathways—that are connected to the diseased area during an acupuncture session. The needles are often left in the patient for 20 to 30 minutes, during which time the patient may feel warm, tingly, or relaxed.

Similar in concept, acupressure uses the fingers, thumbs, or specialized tools to apply hard pressure to certain locations. This little pressure helps reduce the symptoms of CTS by facilitating the passage of energy and releasing muscle tension.

While some CTS sufferers find great relief from acupuncture and acupressure, it's important to speak with a certified professional about your symptoms and medical background before beginning any treatment. They can guarantee that these therapies are in line with your overall treatment strategy and offer tailored advice.

Spinal Alignment And Chiropractic Care

The goal of chiropractic care is to maximize spinal alignment and function to support general health and well-being. It focuses on the interaction between the spine and the nervous system. By treating underlying issues that contribute to nerve compression and dysfunction, chiropractic adjustments may provide relief for people suffering from Carpal Tunnel Syndrome (CTS).

A chiropractor will examine the alignment of the wrists, arms, and spine, with special attention to the neck and upper back, during a chiropractic evaluation for CTS. Subluxations, another name for misalignments, can put pressure on nerves, especially the median nerve, which is implicated in CTS.

To restore optimal alignment and mobility, gentle manipulations of the spine and joints are performed during chiropractic adjustments. These changes may help reduce CTS symptoms like pain, numbness, and weakness by reducing pressure on nerves and enhancing nerve function.

To promote optimal nerve health and lower the chance of a recurrence of CTS, chiropractors may also suggest supplementary therapies like stretching exercises, ergonomic adjustments, and lifestyle modifications in addition to spinal adjustments.

It's crucial to speak with a certified chiropractor who has expertise in treating patients with comparable issues if you're thinking about receiving chiropractic care for CTS. To encourage healing and symptom relief, they can customize a treatment plan to meet your unique requirements and preferences. This plan may include a combination of adjustments and supportive therapies.

Supplements And Herbal Remedies

Supplements and herbal medicines are frequently investigated as complementary therapies for a range of illnesses, including Carpal Tunnel Syndrome (CTS). Certain herbs and nutrients may have anti-inflammatory, analgesic, and nerve-protective qualities that could help people with CTS, despite the paucity of data on their efficacy in treating the condition.

Turmeric is one herb that has drawn interest due to its possible function in the management of CTS. Turmeric's primary ingredient, curcumin, has anti-inflammatory properties that may help lessen swelling and pain related to CTS. It can be administered topically as a cream or ointment or taken orally as a supplement.

Arnica Montana is another herbal treatment that could help with CTS symptoms. This plant-based treatment, which is often applied topically as gels or creams to reduce pain and swelling related to musculoskeletal injuries and diseases like CTS, possesses analgesic and anti-inflammatory qualities.

Supplements that promote nerve function and wellness may also be beneficial to those with CTS, in addition to natural therapies. For instance, vitamin B6 is essential for nerve function and can help lessen symptoms like tingling and numbness in the hands and wrists. Fish oil supplements contain omega-3 fatty acids, which have anti-inflammatory qualities that may help reduce CTS-related discomfort and inflammation.

It's important to speak with a healthcare professional before adding herbal remedies or supplements to your CTS treatment plan, especially if you use any drugs or have underlying medical disorders. They can advise you on possible interactions, and safe and proper usage, and assist you in making decisions regarding your health.

Talking About Alternative Therapies With Medical Professionals

Open and sincere communication is crucial while looking for alternative remedies for Carpal Tunnel Syndrome (CTS) with your healthcare providers. While splinting, corticosteroid injections, and surgery are among the standard treatments for CTS, complementary and alternative therapies including acupuncture, chiropractic adjustments, and herbal remedies may provide more choices for managing and relieving symptoms.

Starting a discussion about alternative therapies with your healthcare professional will assist in guaranteeing that your treatment plan is thorough and customized to your specific requirements and preferences. Your healthcare professional can provide information about the possible advantages and disadvantages of alternative therapies as well as how they might work in tandem or independently with traditional methods.

Be ready to describe your symptoms, medical history, and any prior CTS treatments or therapies you've attempted during these conversations. Your healthcare professional will use this information to evaluate the suitability of alternative therapies and provide recommendations tailored to your unique situation.

It's also crucial to get advice from experts in the field when thinking about CTS alternative treatments. Seek professionals with training and experience in the particular therapy you are interested in, such as herbal medicine, chiropractic adjustments, or acupuncture. They can guarantee that therapies are provided safely and successfully and offer tailored recommendations.

You may confidently investigate alternate therapy for CTS and make well-informed decisions regarding your treatment path by having an open discussion with your healthcare provider and getting advice from trained specialists.

Complementary Therapies: Including Them In CTS Treatment Plans

Complementary therapies can be incorporated into treatment programs for Carpal Tunnel Syndrome (CTS) to provide a comprehensive approach to managing symptoms and enhance overall health.

Acupuncture, chiropractic adjustments, and nutritional supplements are examples of complementary therapies that can be used in addition to more traditional treatments like corticosteroid injections, surgery, and wrist splinting to alleviate CTS symptoms.

Collaborating with a diverse healthcare team is one approach to incorporating complementary medicines into treatment regimens for CTS. Primary care doctors, orthopedic specialists, physical therapists, chiropractors, acupuncturists, and other medical experts who may offer knowledge and direction in their specialized domains may be on this team.

Those with CTS can obtain a wide choice of treatment options catered to their requirements and preferences by speaking with a variety of healthcare professionals.

This cooperative strategy enables individualized treatment that targets the root causes of CTS symptoms and encourages the best possible healing and recuperation.

People with CTS can proactively include alternative therapies into their self-care routines in addition to consulting with healthcare experts.

This could entail using ergonomic work practices to lessen the strain on the hands and wrists, engaging in stress-relieving activities like yoga or mindfulness meditation, and increasing their intake of anti-inflammatory foods and supplements.

Patients can enhance their quality of life and maximize their treatment outcomes by adopting a comprehensive strategy for CTS therapy that incorporates alternative and conventional therapies.

Chronic fatigue syndrome (CTS) symptoms can be more effectively and sustainably managed with proactive self-care and guidance from skilled healthcare providers.

CHAPTER EIGHT

TIPS FOR DAILY ACTIVITIES FOR PEOPLE LIVING WITH CTS

Having Carpal Tunnel Syndrome (CTS) might make it difficult to go about your everyday business. However, efficient symptom management and maintenance of a high quality of life are achievable with the correct accommodations and assistance.

Modifications For Typical Daily Tasks

Making small adjustments to your daily schedule can have a big impact on how well your CTS symptoms are managed. For instance, to lessen wrist strain when cooking, use lightweight tools and utensils. Think about utilizing kitchen appliances that are ergonomic and meant to reduce wrist strain. Divide up cleaning chores into manageable chunks to prevent extended durations of repetitive motion. To lessen the strain on your hands and wrists, choose instruments with bigger grips or handles.

Modify your workstation at work to encourage good wrist alignment and relieve strain on the median nerve. To keep your wrists neutral, place your keyboard and mouse at elbow height. Purchase an ergonomic chair with adequate lumbar support to promote excellent posture and lessen hand and wrist strain.

Utilizing Assistive Technology In CTS Management

To reduce wrist strain and manage CTS symptoms, assistive gadgets might be very helpful. To relieve pressure on the median nerve and lessen pain and tingling, wrist splints can assist in maintaining the wrist in a neutral position. To maintain your wrist in a neutral position while you sleep, think about using a wrist splint. This can help with symptoms and enhance the quality of your sleep.

For those with CTS who have trouble typing or using a mouse, voice recognition software can be a lifesaver. You can lessen the pressure on your wrists and hands while still completing activities quickly by dictating text and speaking commands. Examine several software choices to determine which one best fits your requirements and tastes.

Advice For Operating A Vehicle, Typing, And Other Tasks

It can be painful to drive while you have CTS, especially if you spend a lot of time behind the wheel. A comfortable and ergonomic driving position can be achieved by adjusting the seat and steering wheel to reduce wrist strain. If you want to give your hands some extra cushioning and support, think about utilizing a steering wheel cover with additional padding.

Take frequent breaks to extend your hands and wrists and relax your wrists when typing or using a computer. Use proper typing form by keeping your fingers loose and your wrists straight. To lessen the need for repetitious typing, think about utilizing speech recognition software or keyboard shortcuts.

Activity And Rest Balanced For Healthy Wrists

It's critical to strike the correct balance between rest and activity to manage CTS symptoms and support wrist health. Steer clear of tasks like heavy lifting and repetitive motions that aggravate your wrists. Instead, to increase wrist and hand strength and flexibility, include mild stretches and exercises in your routine.

Pay attention to your body's needs and take pauses when necessary to recuperate. To maintain general wrist health, pace yourself throughout activities to prevent overexertion and give self-care skills like mindfulness, relaxation techniques, and stress management priority.

Asking Friends And Family For Support

It might be difficult to live with CTS, but you don't have to do it alone. Seek out the help of loved ones who can provide understanding, encouragement, and support. Ask for assistance when you need it, and be upfront and honest in communicating your needs.

Joining a support group for people with CTS can help you meet people going through similar things. Talking to others about your experiences, advice, and coping mechanisms can be a great way to get support and validation. Additionally, think about getting advice from medical specialists like occupational or physical therapists, who can offer tailored suggestions and assistance for successfully managing CTS symptoms.

CHAPTER EIGHT

PROSPECTIVE DEVELOPMENTS AND STUDIES IN CTS MANAGEMENT

New Approaches To Treat CTS

The management of carpal tunnel syndrome (CTS) involves an ongoing search for better therapies that reduce symptoms and improve the patient's quality of life.

New therapies present encouraging options for people suffering from pain associated with CTS. The development of minimally invasive techniques is one such breakthrough. Compared to conventional surgery, some methods—like endoscopic carpal tunnel release—need fewer incisions and require shorter recovery periods.

Regular activities can be resumed by patients sooner, which promotes a quicker return to everyday routines.

Regenerative medicine is a field that has seen some fascinating developments recently. For example, stem cell therapy may be able to restore the carpal tunnel's injured tissues.

The objective of this method is to mitigate the symptoms of CTS and encourage tissue regeneration by utilizing the body's healing capabilities.

Although the research is still in its early phases, preliminary findings point to encouraging results, which gives the medical community hope.

Furthermore, pharmacological developments provide fresh approaches to treating CTS symptoms. Pharmaceutical advances accommodate specific patient demands and preferences, ranging from innovative drug formulations to targeted therapy.

Topical treatments, for example, might offer localized comfort by directly addressing the afflicted area.

Furthermore, the goal of pain management innovations such as nerve blocks and sustained-release formulations is to offer less invasive, long-lasting symptom relief.

Additionally, conservative options for the management of CTS are provided by the ongoing evolution of non-invasive therapies. Methods like acupuncture, laser therapy, and therapeutic ultrasound are effective in lowering pain and enhancing functional results. These modalities are essential parts of multimodal treatment approaches that are suited to the specific requirements of each patient. They are frequently supplemented by specially made bracing or splinting.

The field of CTS treatment is constantly changing as a result of breakthroughs in technology and research, giving individuals who are suffering from this crippling illness fresh hope.

Progress In Diagnostic Methods

To successfully manage carpal tunnel syndrome (CTS) and put prompt measures in place to reduce symptoms and stop development, an accurate diagnosis is essential. The way clinicians approach CTS assessment has changed dramatically as a result of advancements in diagnostic tools, which allow for more accurate diagnosis and definition of the syndrome.

The field of imaging modalities is one area of noteworthy progress. For example, high-resolution ultrasound provides a non-invasive, economical way to view the median nerve and evaluate the shape of the carpal tunnel. Dynamic evaluation made possible by real-time imaging enables medical professionals to identify minute variations in the size and movement of nerves.

As a result, patients receive the best possible care, and diagnosis accuracy is increased along with targeted treatment planning facilitation.

Moreover, nerve conduction studies (NCS) and electromyography (EMG) continue to be essential diagnostic methods for CTS evaluation. But as technology developed, these

methods were improved, becoming more sensitive and specific. Sophisticated signal processing methods in conjunction with
advanced EMG protocols allow for the accurate localization of nerve compression sites and the distinction of CTS from other neuropathic disorders. Parallel to this, advancements in NCS techniques enable more precise nerve conduction velocity measurements and the identification of minute anomalies suggestive of CTS.

Furthermore, the amalgamation of artificial intelligence (AI) and machine learning exhibits the potential to transform the diagnosis of CTS. AI systems can help physicians diagnose patients more accurately by evaluating large datasets and spotting complex patterns in patient profiles. AI-powered diagnostic technologies, which range from image recognition to predictive modeling, enhance clinical judgment, expedite the diagnosis process, and lower diagnostic errors.

All things considered, improvements in diagnostic methods enable medical professionals to quickly and precisely identify CTS, opening the door to prompt therapies and better patient outcomes.

Studies On The Prevention Of CTS

To lessen the impact of carpal tunnel syndrome (CTS) and lower its occurrence in at-risk populations, prevention is crucial. Studies devoted to the prevention of CTS provide insight into lifestyle changes, ergonomic treatments, and modifiable risk factors that can be used to avoid the onset or worsening of this incapacitating illness.

Occupational ergonomics is one area of interest in CTS preventive studies. Research examines how ergonomic interventions, equipment modifications, and workplace design affect the prevalence of repetitive strain injuries (CTS) in people who perform repetitive manual tasks. The goal of strategies like ergonomic training programs, workplace ergonomics assessments, and ergonomic guidelines' application is to reduce cumulative stress to the wrist and median nerve while optimizing biomechanics.

Additionally, lifestyle changes are essential for preventing CTS, especially in those with metabolic syndrome or obesity as risk factors. Studies investigate the impact of lifestyle factors, including nutrition, exercise, and stress reduction, on the development of CTS. Weight management plans, exercise routines, and stress reduction methods are a few examples of interventions that support good lifestyle choices and may be useful in reducing the risk of CTS and enhancing general musculoskeletal health.

Furthermore, studies look into the effectiveness of preventive actions aimed at particular high-risk groups. Various research is being conducted to develop customized strategies for reducing the incidence of CTS in various demographic groups. These tactics range from ergonomic interventions for computer users or musicians to customized therapies for pregnant women.

Additionally, the use of technology in CTS prevention research promises to yield novel treatments and tools for individualized risk assessment. Individuals at risk of chronic fatigue syndrome can receive personalized feedback and real-time tracking of biomechanical parameters using wearable devices, ergonomic monitoring systems, and mobile health applications.

Research studies on CTS prevention open the door to proactive interventions and improved musculoskeletal health among groups prone to this syndrome by clarifying modifiable risk variables and viable preventative techniques.

www.ingramcontent.com/pod-product-compliance
Lightning Source LLC
Chambersburg PA
CBHW071840210526
45479CB00001B/220